What Women Want

The Manual for Men

I0448105

By
Amanda Jordan

Table of Contents

Introduction

I want to thank you and congratulate you for downloading the book What Women Want: The Manual for Men.

This book contains proven steps and strategies on how to become truly irresistible to women. You will learn:

- The games women play, why they play them, and how to recognize and avoid them.
- The top 5 traits that women find completely irresistible in a man and how you can learn to embody these traits.
- The things that really turn women on in the bedroom.
- How to be a gentleman and get what you want from a woman by giving her what she wants as well.

Here's an inescapable fact: you will need to broaden your horizons of your understanding of women in order to have more meaningful and long lasting friendships and partnerships with them.

If you do not develop your understanding of what women want, that could potentially lead to a lifelong battle of frustration and loneliness.

It's time for you to become an amazing, confident man who women want to be around, be with, and please!

Chapter 1: Evaluate and Reevaluate What <u>You</u> Want in a Woman

Men and women have been boggling each other's minds since there have been men and women. Even the father of modern psychoanalysis, Dr. Sigmund Freud, went to his death bed without ever really fully understanding the female psyche as much as he would have liked to. In fact, the poor guy was way off, especially when it comes to women in this day and age.

Not so long ago (and even in some instances still today) the structure of society put women in a position to be heavily dependent on men to provide a life for them. It was the norm that men and women each had their roles somewhat neatly laid out for them like a 1950's era sitcom script. However, the roles of men and women in a relationship have continued to evolve as we as a people have, of course.

Luckily, we are living in a society that not only values but also continues to propel itself toward complete gender equality; but the constant evolution of male and female relationships can sometimes naturally bring with it, even more, mystery, confusion, and even frustration.

Any modern woman could simultaneously be looking for a casual relationship, a committed relationship, or any varying degree of both or either. Women already in a committed relationship also want varying degrees of different things, seemingly suddenly or unexpectedly at times while also expecting their significant other to keep up. Deciding factors could be anything from (but certainly not limited to) career to family to the men she encounters, which includes you.

Evaluate What <u>You</u> Want from a Woman and a Relationship

The beginning is always a great place to start, and your encounter with any woman - whether you've been married to someone for thirty years or you're out on the prowl - begins with you. Take stock of what you want and need, regardless of your relationship status. This exercise will help you to gain a better understanding of what women want from you, so pay attention here guys.

While it's healthy to keep a significant other or the prospect of one in mind when planning your future, don't even factor in a particular woman at first here. Just focus on what it is you desire in a woman, relationship, or partner. While you can simply take a mental note, it is advisable to actually write out a list.

Don't worry. It doesn't need to be a novel. Just jot down everything that comes to mind when it comes to what you want and what you need and what you are looking for in a woman and in a relationship with a woman. Don't get too distracted by refining this list just yet - that will come later. You would be surprised how much time and heartache this simple exercise can save you and your partner or future partner. You can put as much or as little time into this as you like. Be mindful of your choices but don't overthink it. It's your life. Make it your list.

- Evaluate what you are looking for in a partner, significant other, what have you. It is so easy to fall for someone who is hot, funny, sweet, mysterious, wealthy, smart, or is a socialite, et cetera when relationships are in their budding phases, and everything is coming up roses. In your list, make sure to include qualities and traits that will endure through the hard times as well. These traits will, of course, overlap a bit, but anyone who has ever dated an extremely beautiful woman for any amount of time will tell you – looks aren't everything. If the going gets tough, you wouldn't want someone to bail on you in your time of need. If you want a gal to stick it out with you through thick and thin, make sure you include in your list such traits as 'good listener,' 'compassionate,' or 'loyal,' to name a few.

- Evaluate what your reasons are for being with or finding a significant other. Really, *really* ask yourself why you are wanting a significant other in your life. Now, it is important to keep in mind that you are by NO means evaluating your current relationship here if you are in one. That will be covered later on in this book. Just ask yourself what YOUR reasons are for wanting to be in a relationship. Are you looking for someone to keep you company only when you happen to be feeling a little lonely, or a relationship of convenience? Are you looking for someone to 'hang out' with – grab a drink or dinner or share an intimate evening with occasionally? Are you looking for 'the one'? Are you looking for a monogamous relationship? Are you looking for a lifetime partner? Are you seeking marriage? Have you already found the love of your life and you are looking to continue to see that relationship grow? So often, both men and women think they want a monogamous, committed, long-term relationship when what they really want is someone for right now, and then maybe the relationship will continue and maybe it won't. Do you care either way, right here, right now? Knowing your own reasons for wanting a relationship or wanting to continue a relationship will set the pace with that special lady because it will help you communicate that to her. If you don't prefer to see your significant other every day, but she wants to spend all of her free time with you, that instance alone could pose some problems down the line and eventually lead to the inevitable breakup. All because you didn't really realize what you wanted in the first place and so were not able to communicate that to her. There are no wrong answers here at all. So go ahead and feel free to be completely and absolutely honest, you owe it to yourself.

- Evaluate what your level of maturity is when it comes to navigating relationships. Maturity does matter a lot whether you want a long-term, lifetime, bed buddy, or anything in between kind of relationship. There will always be those crossroads and obstacles along the way that would challenge even the strongest of commitments at times, but if you happen to be mature enough to know how to handle your relationship, you can make those tough calls and solid decisions which will ensure that your relationship will last. A way to gauge your relationship maturity level is to ask yourself whether or not you are quick to anger or if you get jealous too easily or if you sweat the little things too much – like her leaving a toothbrush out or not managing her time in a way that you like. A mature man knows when to keep fighting for he wants or needs or likes and when just to let it go, without being a doormat. A man who is mature in relationships is okay with losing the battle in order to win the war – the war being you and her against the world, not you against her.

- Evaluate whether or not you yourself are able to differentiate between a good relationship and a bad relationship. A good relationship, whether it is in the confines of family, friendship, work, or a partner, is something that enriches your life and motivates you to keep bettering yourself as a person. A positive relationship will bring about a positive change in your life and will empower you to strive to reach the goals that you set for yourself. A good relationship will nurture the person you are and encourage you to continue to work toward the things in life that will make you happy and will also be the support you need when you happen to fail or make mistakes or are in need of a little extra attention from time to time. Contrary to all of those things, a bad relationship will only serve to drain you of all your positive energy. A bad relationship will bring you down, will consistently make you question your worth as a person, and will also consistently hurt you either physically or emotionally or both. No one should ever stay in a bad relationship, it is extremely unhealthy. A man who stays in bad relationship is basically emitting three things out into the world. While he may not particularly be thinking or feeling these things, this is what everyone around him sees, either consciously or subconsciously. The first is that he doesn't really care all that much about himself or his world. The second thing is that he doesn't believe he is worthy of happiness or love. The third thing that a man who chooses to stay in a bad relationship is doing is essentially giving the woman in the relationship permission to continue to hurt him. Women are not the only victims of this issue. There is no shame in walking away from a toxic relationship. If you feel like you are in one, get out immediately and let it go completely.

- Evaluate whether or not you are really ready for marriage – this evaluation step is for those of you who have not yet tied the proverbial knot. The younger you are, the more it seems like you know everything and the older you get, you come to realize that you don't really know all that much after all right? Whether or not this holds true to you personally, the key to knowing if you are ready for marriage or not is as simple and as complicated as knowing yourself. Some men get into a relationship without marriage ever even factoring into the equation. This is by no means a bad thing at all, just make sure you are aware of where you stand with this and do not be shy about letting your lady know where you stand. Marriage may not be that big of a big deal to some people, but it very well may matter to your girlfriend of three years who wants to get married (finally) and you can't even imagine turning off your gaming console long enough to even talk about marriage, much less actually plan for it. (What was she thinking?! Everything was going so well!) While it is obviously not all your fault, you are partially to blame. You should keep in mind that marriage, or some form of legal coupling is normally the end game of a romantic relationship. That or a breakup. While many women are in no hurry to go rushing down the aisle, it is a wildly romantic gesture that a lot of people keep in the back of their minds. Whether you know you are ready for marriage, not ready for marriage, don't ever want to ever get married ever, or you're just simply unsure, don't go wasting your significant other's time and affections by not being up front. Even an 'I don't know, definitely not right now or in the next few years' is better than nothing. If you're not in a relationship already, before you get into one let your principle on marriage be known. There is no need for this to be 'a talk'. It is simple enough to state this in passing early on, then revisit it once a commitment is being made.

Evaluate What You Want in a Woman

Now that you have a somewhat complete evaluation of what you want from a woman and why you want it, you now need to spend some time refining and reevaluating what you've written. Or what you think you want. Again, this doesn't necessarily have to be a long drawn out affair.

Often times during this reevaluation process, though, even men who consider themselves to be very self-aware have had to admit that seeing something that they thought they wanted or didn't want actually written down on paper just simply made them scratch their heads at their own choices. If something just doesn't look right or makes you think twice when you read it, spend a bit of time rethinking your reasoning. Ask yourself if that list is an accurate representation of yourself and what you are really looking for.

Make sure you don't do yourself the disservice of either including or omitting items just because you think someone else may approve or disapprove. Remember that this is only going to work for you if you are completely honest with yourself, and there are no wrong answers.

While the following is by no means an exhaustive list, here are some tips to get the wheels in your mind turning and to help you in the reevaluation process:

- What is your favorite item on your list? Why? What on your list would make you the happiest if you had that with a woman and/or in a relationship? People often do what they think others want them to do, which is natural human behavior – it is part of what keeps society intact, but if your favorite item on the list is a raunchy sex fest, so be it. If it's cuddling up with the cutest bookworm you've ever seen to have a nerdy movie marathon, go for it. From having a family and growing old with someone to one night stands with numerous women, just be honest with yourself about what you want and WHY you want it. This will make your life so much easier, both in the here and now and also in the long run. Whichever your favorite item on the list may be, make sure you look for that quality in a woman – you will be doing what you love and love what you are doing day in and day out.

- Does one item on your list make mention of being with a woman who wants to be happy? Of course, there are varying degrees of happiness, but surrounding yourself with people who actually like being happy as opposed to keeping company with the emotional vampires of the world is a key ingredient to your own happiness, especially when it comes to a significant other.

- Does your list include items that will help you to get closer to achieving your personal goals in life? For example, if one of your life's goals is to have a career that calls for a lot of travel, how does what you want in a woman fit into that? Did you include the adjective 'supportive' in your list?

- It is imperative that we as people take the time to just live in the moment every once in a while. You have an unexpected afternoon off. Do you take a walk in the park, feed some ducks, and strike up a conversation with an elderly man playing chess instead of heading straight home to the TV? It can be really enlightening to move outside of your normal bubble or do something completely spontaneous. Are you looking for a sense of adventure in a woman?

- Arguments and fights happen. They are part of life and actually bring a couple closer together when resolved maturely. Did you make sure to include things like sense of humor, humble, and forgiving?

- Health is important to us all, though something that healthy people usually end up taking for granted. Is good health included in the list of qualities you're looking for in a lady?

- Downtime is absolutely necessary for everybody at some point in any relationship. Often times with a woman, this can be a really rewarding opportunity to solidify your relationship in a low-key, comfortable way. Did you include your desire for her to share the same downtime activities as you do?

Evaluating Your Current Relationship

This is not as life altering or detrimental to your current relationship as you may be thinking. This section is mainly included because men all too commonly make the biggest mistake that is possible to make in a relationship. This mistake is made over and over and over countless times by men all over the world. You're probably thinking 'cheating,' but this is a precursor to cheating - they evaluate the woman instead of the relationship.

Do not do this. Men tend to make this horrifying mistake most often when confronted with a new impending heavy responsibility such as marriage or a new baby. It cannot be stressed enough here guys – don't cheat on the woman that is about to, or just gave birth to, your child. She deserves more than that from you. While you may be feeling neglected, and rightfully so – weddings and pregnancies are all about the woman – absolutely nothing will ever mend the hurt that is caused by that betrayal. You do not want to do that to the mother of your child or to yourself.

Enough said. Getting back to the main point here, men tend to evaluate the woman when looking for reasons to either continue to be with her or to break it off. This is a normal knee jerk reaction, albeit an unhealthy and unfortunate one. The detriment in this instance is that a man can usually find someone who is any combination of better looking, younger, wealthier, more ambitious or well read, et cetera, but the real question is whether or not you are happy with your relationship, bottom line.

It is easy to find fault in a person. It is more difficult to find fault in something that you yourself are responsible for as well. If you're in one of the best relationships you've ever had, count yourself lucky. People go their whole lives without finding happiness in a relationship. Evaluating your current relationship can actually be really healthy and proactive as well. You could ask yourself if both you and she are getting what is needed from a relationship. A "no" or "I don't know" answer is simply an opportunity to reconnect with your special lady and communicate that you care about her happiness as well as your own.

Doing this will always score you major points. Depending on the delivery, it is possible that this could turn into an argument. If this happens, remain calm. Take the high road and simply let her know that you just wanted to check in and have a meaningful conversation – because you care – and that it's up to her to do her part in having a successful conversation about your relationship. Just to recap, do not evaluate your significant other, evaluate the relationship you have together.

Chapter 2: Game On! The Tests and Mind Games Women Use

Let's face it; we have all been guilty of it at one time or another – playing mind games with someone just because we can. While testing each other and pushing boundaries in a relationship is totally normal, playing mind games, however, is not okay.

It cannot be stressed enough how much this manipulative, bullying behavior should have absolutely zero place in your relationship, whether it comes from her, you, or both of you. Purposely toying with someone's mind or emotions just because you can is nothing to brag about. Unfortunately some men and women both find this behavior not only acceptable on some level but something to have an impish good laugh over when with friends.

Why Do We Engage in Mind Games?

The biggest reason people put up with manipulative mind games, especially ones known to cause pain and negativity, is simply because they are afraid of losing the attention or affections of the person being manipulative.

How to Recognize the Tests and Mind Games Women Use the Most

Do women play mind games and test men? You bet they do. Men do these things as well, and just as skillfully, but it seems that women resort to playing mind games more often, in order to level out the playing field or gain the upper hand altogether. Sometimes it is a simple matter of harmless flirting or subconscious boundary testing.

Then there are those times that you know she is messing with you just because she can or to get her way. While light, playful little games can be a whole lot of fun when getting to know someone, or keep a relationship fresh and interesting, the games that come into play within a power struggle can be really harmful.

Can you tell the difference between these situations? The following is a list of the most common mind games the ladies play, in no particular order.

1. **We need to talk -** It is quite possible that every man on earth has heard this at one point or another in his life. These four words can make even the manliest and most confident of men quake in their boots and want to retreat to the deepest

cave on the planet. If or when you hear this you should pay attention to when she is choosing to say this to you and how she is saying it. That will be the difference between her making a power move by playing mind games or just needing to talk to you.

(a) Does she say it in front of other people? Mind game. She wants other people to know that you are in trouble. **She wants your immediate attention and the attention of the people around you.** This is in order to manipulate you into usually taking her aside and her having your undivided attention. You could calmly let her know that there are better and healthier ways of getting attention. **She doesn't need to make a fool of you or herself in the process.**

(b) Does she *always* say it at a time when she knows you are busy with something that does not involve her, such as watching a game or show on TV, work project, or hanging out with your friends or your kid(s)? Especially if this happens consistently, she is playing this card to its fullest mind game potential, and **she knows *exactly* what she is doing**. If she hardly ever does this, don't worry about it as much. It's the consistency that is the most telling. Yet again, she is jealous of your attention and is unsure of how to get it in a healthy manner or is being impatient. Either way, you need to nip this in the bud.

(c) Does she say it with her hand on her hip, head cocked to one side and a scowl on her face? Mind game. This particular instance usually also takes place in front of other people, unfortunately. **This charade is played out to make you look like the bad guy.** No matter what you may have done or not done, the point is that it is important to set a clear boundary here. **Let her know calmly but firmly that you are just not interested in engaging in manipulative behavior and if she wants to keep hanging out/continue the relationship, she must make the choice to no longer engage in that behavior either.**

(d) However, if the lady in your life comes to you in earnest, wanting to resolve an issue that's been on her mind, she will choose to let you know in a tactful, respectful, loving manner when no one else is around, even if she does choose to use those four unfortunate words. If she does feel the need to let you know she wants to talk while you are around other people, she will choose to do so quietly and without putting on any kind of a show. There is absolutely nothing wrong with setting boundaries early on. If a lady knows that you're not into manipulation and mind games, she will consciously avoid them if she is interested in you. Bottom line, if you want your lady to be straight up and honest with you, be straight up and honest with her, she can handle it.

2. **Playing hard to get.** This particular test normally falls under the "harmless" category. **This is usually a tool women use only to protect themselves, not to purposely mess with you.** What is she protecting herself from? The one night stand type of guys who troll around in bars and other places ladies are known

to frequent. Pretty much all women play hard to get, at least from time to time. This is instinctual in women who are looking for a bit more than just a quick romp between the sheets. Those of you men who are not looking for anything more than that, there's your queue to back off and try to hook up with someone else. If you hit on a lady for the first time, let's say, in a bar and she doesn't immediately respond to you, you're used to that right? It happens. So here is the next important question. What do you do next? Do you go hit on the very next lady who catches your eye? If so, you just successfully reiterated why she played hard to get in the first place. If you are actually interested in getting to know her and she sees you hitting on someone 20 feet away, any self-respecting woman would have some kind of inner dialogue at that point, somewhere along the lines of, "Phew! Dodged that bullet." You just blew it. **It is wildly courageous and respectable for someone to approach a complete stranger and try to make some sort of connection.** Women admire that, but they have also heard every line in the book. If you get a flat out no, it's time to move on. Sometimes though, a woman just needs to know that she is special to you. Why should she want to talk to you when she was perfectly happy minding her own business? Give her a reason. Make her laugh, but do not even think about attempting to make a sexual joke. This type of lady is most likely looking for a gentleman of sorts, meaning manners guys. **If she states something like she thinks she is just going to sit and chill for a little while, that may be an invitation to come back around a little later.** This invitation doesn't mean you've got it made, but it does mean that she is at least somewhat interested. In speaking to you. When you come back around, do not invade her space. Keep a physical distance. Make eye contact, but do not stare at her or check her out. Offer to buy her a drink or ask what she recommends. Make small talk, very small talk. Listen to her. Respond to her and ask her if she is going to be hanging around much longer. You can take it from there. This approach will only work if you are genuinely interested in more than a one night stand.

3. **The baiting game. AKA, "Does this make me look fat?"** By no means whatsoever, are you to ever answer this question directly. Even a woman would tell you that. When a woman asks you a question about her physical appearance, less is more. Like, less as in nothing at all. If you don't want to address the fact that she is baiting you – or asking you a question whose answer you will be judged on - then you will be subjected to this type of manipulation for as long as that relationship lasts. Women use this baiting technique for all sorts of things. For example, let's say you're in a fairly new relationship and your lady loves to dye her hair frequently. She knows that your ex was a redhead. She may ask you something as vague as what color you think she should dye her hair. You will probably stammer a bit before answering with something to the effect of I don't know. At this point, she will then ask if you think she should dye her hair red. See where this is going? If you say anything resembling a yes, you may be in for it. A safe answer for these types of things is to ask her if she would like you to pick up a hairstyle mag so she can look at it. **She**

should not be setting you up to fail. Not cool. Let her know that gentlemen. Do not take the bait by reacting to her. Over time, this will lead to her resenting you and finding you unattractive altogether, because she will perceive you as being weak and unable to stand up for yourself by not being able to stand up to her.

4. **The waiting game.** There are two major ways that women play mind games by making you wait. Before we get into that, let's first touch on when you've finally exchanged numbers and you're both electric with the anticipation of sending text messages and talking on the phone. Only, she isn't texting you back. Why? Ladies do not wish to appear to be any more eager or clingy than men do, but there is a chance that she is not actually playing mind games. First of all, if you have only sent a text message that could've been sent to anyone (include her name guys. Ask how she is doing. Tell her you can't wait to see her again and suggest a specific action like going to dinner), she will be less likely to respond. I mean, how would you respond to a text stating,

"Weird day. Can't wait to hit the gym." Really dude? That text is way **too vague and is way too impersonal**. Instead try something like "Hey (woman's name), how has your day been? I had a weird day today so I can't wait to hit the gym. Can I call you after?" Wouldn't you be more likely to respond to a text that included your name and asked you a question? The first text just comes off as thoughtless and lazy. That first text could've been meant for one of your guy friends for all she knows. That having been said, try going that little tiny bit of an extra mile and actually dial her number. Call her. Text messages are basically tiny emails. They are noncommittal and can be sent to anyone. A phone call, however, lets her know that you wanted to actually speak to her, right then and there. If you're still not getting any responses at all after shooting her a few texts messages and leaving a couple of voicemails, it's time to stop trying (a few usually refers to 3, and a couple refers to 2, just to be clear). If she hits you up then game on, but if not you've done your part.

(a)The first way that women play mind games by making you wait is they purposely don't respond to texts or calls because **they do not want to appear to be needy or clingy**. If you are getting concerned or are about to give up after multiple attempts, tell her so. **You can actually tell women the truth, they won't die.** In fact, they will probably view you as refreshing and trustworthy. Women may also cancel last minute. This is common with brand new relationships. A lot of women have damn good reasons, but they sure aren't about to tell you that they just started their period a few days early so they're not feeling especially social. Or that their day just ran a bit long and they don't have time to get ready like they wanted to. Or that they're just plain broke and are waiting for payday just in case. Don't take it as a dig unless it keeps happening and she doesn't make any plans to reconnect.

(b)The second way a woman plays mind games by making you wait is by purposely making you wait when you come to pick them up, meet them at a restaurant or bar, whatever, in order to **build anticipation**. Not only women use this, but it is definitely widely used by women.

Again, the wait could be due to having to run to the nearest store to buy pantyhose because she just got a huge ugly run in hers. Either way, if this occurs often, it is something that should be addressed. You could even sweetly say something along the lines of her being worth the wait but maybe next time she could be on time.

5. **Playing dumb.** There are only two reasons for a woman to play dumb.

6. (a)The first reason is really patronizing and placating to men, but some women find that it is necessary to dumb themselves down when in the company of men, and specifically, their man. Their reasoning for this is that men tend to become intimidated and are turned off by intelligent women.

(b) The second reason that women choose to dumb themselves down for men is to **manipulate men into doing things for them.** While this could be construed as simply being helpful, the odds are that she is perfectly capable of reaching that top shelf with the footstool she hides when you come over, and she can also put together furniture. If you find yourself in this situation, and being the gentleman that you are, it doesn't bother you to help out, you need to address the fact that she feels the need to play dumb in order to get her way. This is a disservice to both her gender and to your relationship. All she has to do is ask, right? Right.

7. **Withholding sex.** This may be perhaps one of the worst mind games women tend to play, with devastating and lasting consequences. As such, not as many women choose to partake in this vile behavior. **For the sake of clarity, this in no way refers to women who *choose* not to have sex** because they're exhausted, menstruating, etc., okay? It is absolutely anyone's prerogative to say no to sex at any time in any relationship. So how can you tell if she is withholding sex to manipulate you? This one is really easy. She will use it as a bargaining chip to get something that she wants, and will only have sex with you after you have accomplished getting her what she wants, and exactly to her liking. Be very wary of these women. If a woman has chosen to enter a sexual relationship with a man

and then all of a sudden starts using sex as a bargaining chip, this changes the unspoken agreement of a sexual relationship and can cause a lot of confusion and frustration. When a woman withholds sex, she is withholding part of the relationship. **By doing this, she is essentially holding your relationship hostage until her demands are met. Don't negotiate with your little relationship terrorist.** Women love sex as much as men do. Absolutely address this issue as head-on as you can muster. Let her know she is sabotaging your entire relationship and not respecting you as a man, or human being for that matter.

8. **Reverse psychology.** Ah yes, the mind game most widely used by women predominantly. Have you ever noticed that a woman is upset and actually asked her what's wrong, only to get the short, cold answer of, "fine."? **Obviously, she is not fine, but why does she expect you to know what is wrong if she refuses to talk about it?** Further questioning in this instance often leads to an awkward outburst of some kind,

usually involving tears. Another good example of a woman using reverse psychology is when **she wants you to do one thing but suggests you do the opposite**. For example, let's say you and she have a dinner date planned for a weekend night. It's nothing special, really just dinner. A day before your planned date, you find out some old buddies will be in town for that night only. So you bring it up to her and explain that you'd really like to reschedule. She may say something like, "Sure. You should go and hang out with your friends", when she really means, "Are you kidding me?! I guess I don't really mean that much to you". This is usually accompanied by some sort of argument the next time she sees you after you have hung out with your friends. Don't coddle her, but let her know how you feel about her. If possible, make it up to her in some way, something as simple as rescheduling immediately. Immediately as in before you break the news that you need to break the date. If you have a plan in mind, like you made a reservation at a spot she's been wanting to go to, for instance, you'll have a better shot at her hurt feelings being assuaged and avoiding this awkward situation altogether. If she continues using this mind game, you must stand up for yourself and your relationship. Set a boundary by telling her what your boundaries are in this area. **Let her know that you would like a relationship that is not manipulative and you will uphold your end of that bargain as well.**

9. **The silent treatment.** The silent treatment is part of a pattern called the **demand-withdraw pattern** and is caused by a combination of hurt feelings and the inability or unwillingness to proactively communicate. Men tend to use the silent treatment to respond to what they consider nagging. Women tend to use this mind game a lot when in the midst of a fairly large disagreement. While it is just a good solid practice to hold your tongue if you have nothing nice to say, she should at least say that much. If the woman in your life chooses the silent treatment as a form of regular 'communication,' **she is trying to manipulate you into feeling guilty, feeling as hurt as she is feeling, and**

into making a huge apology met with flowers and candy, etc. Current collective research on this subject has actually proven that **giving your partner the silent treatment is the fastest way to lead your relationship to a breakup or divorce**. Unfortunately, the silent treatment is one of the most widely used responses in relationship conflict. No wonder nobody stays together.

Chapter 3: Taking the High Road – Being a Nice Guy without Being a Doormat

So when do you take the high road? The short answer is always. It is important for you to strive to take the high road at all times. It can be all too easy and even somewhat gratifying to hurt someone who has hurt you.

All across the globe men and women struggle with periods of upset, difficult conversations, painful discoveries and more. When someone becomes upset or angry, they may often feel the need to lash out, shut down, seek revenge, or explode. Staying calm, cool and collected is often the last thing we human beings want to do when we are hurt or angry.

Sometimes a person may lash out in order to simply because another person pain so that person will know what it feels like to get hurt. Other times a person may lash out as a simple knee-jerk reaction. Regardless of why we as human beings tend to lash out when hurt, we can all understand the urge to want to do so.

The bottom line, though, is that "losing it" on someone in reaction to that person saying hurtful things, or on a spouse or significant other because of their cheating ways, or on a co-worker for jeopardizing your job—will not ever actually serve you well. The last thing you really want to do is make life more difficult for yourself by reacting to the extremes. When you are able to respond to the most difficult circumstances with calm strength and grace, you will heal faster and ultimately feel better about yourself and the world around you. Basically when it comes to handling difficult moments, always try to be mindful of the importance of taking the high road - even though those around you may choose to behave atrociously.

5 Reasons for a Man to Take the High Road:

1. When a man is able to react calmly and with integrity in the face of someone else's choice to engage in hurtful behavior, he will feel empowered, internally strong, and psychologically healthy.

2. When a man chooses to freak out in reaction to someone else's freak out, that person will completely ignore what he is trying to tell them and will only think, "You think I'm crazy – ha - look at you." A poor choice in behavior will get in the way of the other person recognizing their own poor choice in behavior.

3. When a man chooses to react to hurtful or erratic behavior by acting like an unstable person, people around him will view him as a crazy person. When a man responds with integrity, however, others will begin to view the other person as the unstable and unhealthy one instead of him. Be the good guy.

4. When you stoop to the other person's level, you are not true to your own self. You can take the high road with the knowledge that the poor behavior of others is certainly NOT a go-ahead for your own poor behavior.

5. When you are able to stay calm even in the most difficult of moments, you completely avoid the 'over-reactive hangover.' There's no shame, regret, self-hatred, or embarrassment about what you did. It's then easy to feel good about being you and hold your head up high.

Taking the high road really just means to be mindful of acting with integrity at all times - not just the good times. Harming another person whether it is physical, emotionally, or spiritually, is completely without integrity, even when responding to lies, an affair, or manipulations.

Do not try to stoop to some else's level and then claim that your behavior is okay and warranted - it's not. Remember to remain respectful, set limits for yourself, take care of yourself first and then decide how you are going to interact in such a way that you are both respectful of yourself and respectful of the humanity of the other person. This will ensure that you avoid the horrible feeling of the 'over-reactive hangover.' Keep in mind that even though seeking revenge or going off on a person may feel great at the moment, that feeling never lasts forever.

Here is a challenge: If you happen to be struggling with someone else's hurtful behavior, take a step back and try to examine the situation more objectively. Take a deep breath, calm your heart rate down, and be daring enough to go ahead and take that high road. Have it set in your mind to refuse to act like a man who is raging or out of control? Once you have settled yourself, you will be able to then react with a calm inner strength and a sense of grace. If you choose to do this, you will inevitably feel much better for it and will be able to hold your head high knowing you did the right thing for yourself and didn't put any added negativity out into the world.

Be a Gentleman, Not a Doormat

There is never a good time or reason to be a doormat. Nobody ever likes that guy, ever. You do not have to be a doormat in order to be a nice guy. A gentleman first and foremost takes care of himself, mainly because he knows that if he is not at his best (or somewhat close to it), he will be less effective in his duties and relationships. Gentlemen, taking care of yourself first includes ensuring that you are not being taken advantage of or walked on. There is a fine line between being a nice, generous guy and being a complete sucker.

A doormat is a man who bends over backward to please his woman - one who does the things he thinks are necessary in order to try to make his woman happy, no matter how badly she treats him. Here are 8 red flags that you are being used as a doormat by the woman or women in your life.

1.   She gives you 'crumbs' and you pretend that you are perfectly okay with that. Is she just texting you once a week to keep you hanging around, making sure you are still there waiting for her? She may just be stringing you along to keep you as her side dish, and not her main course. Essentially, you have become her backup plan. She is only making sure you are still available on Saturday night, just in case nothing better comes along. You have got to learn about your own boundaries so that you can get the love that you want and the respect that you deserve.

2.   She texts you at the last minute to meet up - and you actually go! She does not even bother to call but instead sends you a text to make a date at 8 PM on a Saturday night. Don't do it, unless you really stress how lucky she is that you didn't have other plans and tell her that you need more of a heads up in the future, or if you have seen each other seriously for a while. Odds are, she's just short on cash and needs you to be her sugar daddy for the night anyhow.

3.   You offer to do things for her that she could and should be doing for herself. Seriously men, if you're not living together, don't even consider offering to pick up her feminine hygiene products or what have you. If she is so busy that she cannot find time to pick them up herself, she has a plethora of other options such as friends, coworkers, classmates; the list goes on.

4.   You take her out to dinner three days a week. This is not to be confused with going out together. In this instance, we're talking specifically about you the man, paying for her dinner by yourself. If you're taking her out to dinner every night and paying for everything, you're training yourself and her that you will be setting yourself up for her expecting you to continue to do this for the entirety of your relationship.

5.   Do you allow her to come over at 3 AM after she's been out drinking? If she is drunk texting you to hang out at this point in her evening, beware: you've become her booty call. While that may not be the worst thing in the world at the time, if you are looking for a relationship, that kind of behavior will only serve to hurt you in the not so long run.

6.   You accept it when she is consistently late to your dates. If she's a few minutes late, give her a break of course, but if you have gone out three or four times and she's always at least half an hour late, you are setting yourself up for becoming a doormat that much more every time it happens.

7.   She leaves or asks you to leave after having sex. Again, this can be a godsend for some guys, but for a man interested in an actual relationship with a woman, this is certainly one of the worst ways to avoid feeling like her doormat. If you happen to enjoy hanging out with or lying next to your lover after sex, she needs to know that this is important to you.

8.   She talks about her sexual conquests in front of you. You are not one of her sorority sisters, and you really do not need her to be telling you about all of the so-called notches on her bedpost.

When it comes to your personal boundaries, make sure you clearly express them. Decide what is acceptable to you and what is unacceptable to you in that relationship. We are all different, but there is absolutely no reason for you to ever be any woman's doormat, even if she's the wealthiest, most beautiful lady you've ever met.

5 Differences Between Being a Nice Guy and Being a Doormat

1. A nice guy is first respectful of himself. This can easily be the biggest perception difference between being a nice guy and being a doormat. If you allow a woman to consistently walk all over you, and you never present your own opinion, you never disagree with her, you never make new suggestions because you are afraid of being outside of your own comfort zone, then it will appear to her as though you do not respect yourself, whether that happens to be true or not.

A nice guy gets that he has his own identity in a relationship as well as his own life for a reason and he can bring his own unique suggestions and interests to the table in a relationship. A nice guy has enough respect for himself, his relationship, and his partner to say no and set those necessary boundaries.

A guy who lets himself become a doormat will believe, however falsely, that if he brings any of his boundaries up it will make too many waves and she will get mad or annoyed, so he just simply lives his life smiling and nodding. Ugh.

2. A nice guy is confident in himself. This pretty much goes hand in hand with #1 but is so important it is well worth its own mention. Notice the word arrogance is not used, but confidence. The biggest reason why some men win and some men lose at the dating game is really their confidence or lack thereof. It does take a fair amount of confidence to initiate any interaction with a woman you do not know.

It takes confidence to make your move. It takes confidence to tell her of your feelings for her. It takes confidence to be secure enough within yourself and your masculinity to be romantic without feeling like you have to sacrifice your masculinity. Any guy who would be considered a doormat very rarely or never displays this confidence.

Your confidence as a man will be your foundation for success not only in relationships but also in life as a whole. Work on this first, and then move forward.

3. A nice guy will show his intentions with respect. This is a huge issue. A lot of the time guys are a bit nervous about making a move or stating their intent towards a woman they care about on some level. The things that go through the minds of most men are things such as - what will happen if she says no? Would we lose our friendship? Will it be awkward now?

After hesitating for so long and questioning it to death, they just never get around to telling that lady friend just how they feel. When a man perpetuates this bad habit but remains friends with the woman he is interested in, she will eventually only see him as a platonic man in her circle of friends who she feels she hang out with like one of the girls.

Women love having men as friends that they are able to interact with the same way they do with their friends who are women. This is what is referred to as the friend zone. Now, this may not appear to be so bad at first because she is showing you some attention, but when you as the man in this instance have a strong desire to be more intimate with said woman, it is absolute torture. A nice man can still be nice and make his intentions known to a woman.

Whether it is placing your hand on her knee or shoulder to see whether or not she reflects your body language, small compliments to see how she responds, or just stepping up to finally ask her out, ladies are no more mind readers than men are. You have to take the risk here and just do it.

You don't have to be the bad boy type in order for her to fall for you either. Nice guys get amazing girlfriends, just like the bad boys. Muster the courage to take it up a notch and take the next step. If she happens to turn you down, then chalk it up to knowing where her boundaries lie with you, at least at the moment, before you become any more invested emotionally.

4. A nice guy isn't overbearing. It is true that a man should put in a consistently solid effort to ensure that the partner in his life feels loved, special, and beautiful. There is a huge difference though between showing someone affection and then smothering them until they feel suffocated. She should be a large part of your life, but certainly not the whole thing.

If you insist on spending every spare second with her or follow her around like a little puppy dog, she will start to feel like you are emotionally suffocating her and she will feel the need to get away from you as quickly as possible. You need to make sure that you give your girl some space.

Respect her boundaries and give her some time to miss you. Additionally, she wants you to have your own hobbies, dreams, passions, and ambitions. She does not want you just to hitch yourself to her passions, just as you do not want her to hitch herself to yours.

5. A nice guy sticks to his boundaries. Both men and women have a tendency to inherently push whatever limits they can until they hit a wall. If you don't understand this, just watch a child whose parents don't intervene when the child is running amok. The behavior will only continue, and it will get worse.

The same goes for most people as adults. If you do not set boundaries for yourself in your relationship, you will constantly be self-sacrificing, and your partner will never be able to develop enough of the respect for you as a man that is necessary in order to see you as a possible romantic interest.

We can all work together to change the common misconception that nice guys always finish last because that is certainly not the case. Doormats do.

Men who voluntarily choose to sacrifice their own sense of self just to try to gain the approval of a woman (or anyone at all) will always finish last. We have all known people who lose sight of their individuality because they are too caught up in trying to please someone else.

Those men finish last. The truth is you don't necessarily have to be just a good guy or only a bad boy; you can absolutely be any varying degrees of both. Challenge her, empower her, seduce her, yes; but also honor, love, and value her.

Chapter 4: Five Things That Make You Irresistible to Women

Have you ever wondered what makes a woman decide to choose you, specifically? There are specific things about men that women absolutely adore. As a matter of fact, they can't help it. Have you ever seen a woman going absolutely gaga eyes over a certain guy, while you are left wondering what it is that is so special about him? The chances are solid that he had at the very least, one or more of these traits. The truth is that even one of these traits, when properly developed, would have women completely falling over themselves just to be around you. Imagine if you could combine at least two of these things! You would literally become absolutely irresistible to women. Saving the best for last, here are five things that make a man irresistible to a woman.

1. **Listening. Really listening** - The honest truth, as we all know by now, is that women really love to talk. That is how they make sense of the world, it seems. The secret here is to be interested and not focused on being interesting. In other

words, you will build attraction by paying closer attention to her and by utilizing active listening. It is not about you, how much money you make, what you drive, who you know, or what experiences you've had. Once she knows you are actually listening, she will start to ask you questions about yourself. When you're first getting to know a woman, the conversation should be about 75% her and about 25% you. That translates into you spending most of your time listening. Be genuinely interested in her instead of talking about yourself and trying to make yourself seem interesting. Even though women are happy to listen to you, a part of them isn't satisfied with the conversation when they don't get a chance to talk about themselves as much as they would like. This does not necessarily mean that women are egocentric and vain, this is just how women get to know men. How well you listen will directly correlate to getting her number, getting a first date, making her your girlfriend, and so on. If you listen well by giving your full, undivided attention, your woman will know that you are interested *and* interesting. Ask her questions about what she is saying. Make eye contact. Don't check out that hottie walking past you. **The more you listen, which helps her to navigate her own feelings and experiences, the more she will be interested in you** or continue to be interested in you. Follow this advice, and before you know it, she just can't wait to tell all of her friends what a great listener you are and how she hasn't had a *real* conversation like that with a guy in a long time. At some point in your conversation, she will definitely comment on what a great listener you are and how interesting the conversation has been. Then you know you have officially arrived at being a great listener in her eyes. Good job. Now she will want to talk with you more and find out more about you.

2. **Proving that you are trustworthy and faithful -** Do what you say you are going to do. Be where you say you are going to be. This is not because she needs to know where you are at all times, by any means. It just means that she needs to know that your word means something so that she doesn't have to worry so much all the time. Women are natural worriers. Don't needlessly make her worry about

whether or not you are who you say you are, and if she is going to get hurt by yet another man who chooses to lie over honesty, cheating over fidelity; you get the picture. A woman's world revolves around her relationships. So naturally, if a woman has any reason to doubt you at your word, it is going to make her worry that a part of her world may choose to leave her. Women have an extremely real natural built-in fear that you are going to leave. So it puts them much more at ease if they feel they can trust you and have some peace of mind knowing that you have no interest in jumping ship so easily. That is why many women value marriage so greatly. One major thing they want to be able to believe is that you are not looking to leave them, but that does not necessarily mean you have to marry your special lady to ensure that she feels secure. You have the opportunity to display acts of faithfulness and trustworthiness every day. Instead of ogling that hot blond with massive breasts walking past you, as difficult as that may be, just keep your eyes on her - and don't even try to steal a glance. Even if you think your lady doesn't notice, she does. Also, just keep your promises. Just some food for thought here, most promises don't actually include the words, "I promise..." okay? Again, be where you say you'll be when you say you will be there, and do what you say you'll do. If you feel like she is nagging you, it's probably because you have not kept your word on something. If a woman feels like she can't trust you to do a simple thing like do what you say you are going to do, that makes her doubt other things you have told her, like how much you care about her, that she has no reason to be jealous of that girl you flirt with at work, et cetera. Honesty is the best policy here. If you feel you need to lie to your partner, this usually means that your actions may be in need of correction.

3. **Showing her your talents and passions.** No one ever really wonders why rock stars have women flocking to them, right? There are very few things that happen to be sexier and more attractive to women than men who are really talented and/or passionate about something (and no, video games don't really work here, guys). When a man has a talent that he really enjoys, his energy is engrossed in it, and it is wildly infectious

to the ladies. Women love to see a man using his talents, if for no other reason than to just make himself a happier, more rounded individual. In the same way, when a man is focusing all of his energy on something he is passionate about, and when a woman sees that passion, she is drawn to him like a moth to the flame. You don't even have to be particularly good at your endeavor (although it certainly doesn't hurt), as long as your energy goes into it. If you don't really have any talents and aren't really passionate about anything, being passionate about finding your passion and hidden talents could be that one thing that makes a particular woman see you in a new light and start finding that she's unable to resist you. As a side note, it is strongly suggested to try volunteering for a nonprofit in your community if you're searching for your passion. Enlightenment hides in some really unexpected places sometimes, and women love men who do things for other people.

4. **Exhibiting charisma and charm.** Being naturally charismatic and charming are amazing traits to possess, but those traits don't always come so easily to every

man. Those traits give a man that special edge which enables a woman to feel like she is something really special and that you are truly a real gentleman. The word gentleman itself is, in essence, describing a man who is charming and has chosen to become gentle, affable, pleasing, well mannered, et cetera. This does not mean that he has lost his masculinity whatsoever. It really just means that he has become able to control himself and conduct himself in a positive, evolved manner. This, men, is what women want. It's all about being smart, about possessing a sense of sophistication on some level, about being somewhat well groomed and living a life that is well worth living. Utilizing charisma and charm takes practice but here are some really basic starting points to get you heading in the right direction:

(a) Use your manners! Even using basic manners goes a long way with the ladies. Say please and thank you. Exercise kindness to the people who serve you food and beverages when you are out with her. Excuse yourself politely if you need to leave her company while out.

(b) Compliment her. Do not even bother with those dime a dozen throw away compliments. When complimenting a woman, use her name in the sentence. A simple formula to giving genuine, great compliments that work every single time is something like this: (Woman's name) I like (thing) because (your reason) [pause] (ask her a question about thing). For example, "Jessica, I really like your hair down because it's so long and wavy. Where do you get it done?" Simple enough.

(c) Chivalry is not dead. Being chivalrous is definitely still in, even with the most feminist, modern woman. It never actually went away, and women find it very attractive whenever a man chooses to be chivalrous. Chivalry seems to have skipped a generation or two, so when you are chivalrous, women are going to take notice. Whenever you are chivalrous, you will stand out far and above most other men. Open the door for her, pull her chair out, and ask her politely but decisively if you can order the wine for the table. Just make sure you don't overdo it with a lot of big show.

Quietly, quickly, eye contact. If you open the door for her but do not make any eye contact, your attempt at chivalry will be dead in the water because it can come off as too cold and like it's a chore you're just trying to get through.

5. **Confidence**. Last but most importantly of all, what all women are attracted to a confident man. Confident men really are sexy as hell in a woman's eyes. Confidence stems from a man feeling secure within himself, and it takes confidence in order to be direct. To women, it is obvious that these two things go hand in hand. There is a reason that you have probably heard all five of these issues brought up, and most likely more than once, when it comes to what women really want in a man. Many single women trying to navigate the dating scene read dating advice columns and respond to these columns with their frustrations regarding how tough the dating world can actually be. The most common complaint across the board among these single women is that men *lack confidence*. Indirect, overly passive men, who are not open about their thoughts or feelings, have no set plan,

zero clear intentions, and make dating feel exhausting and awkward as opposed to being fun like it should be. A woman does not want to have to guess at what you feel because she doesn't want to have to feel uncertain in the relationship. If you are direct and confident while other men remain passive and unclear, there is no contest – you'll already be way ahead of the curve in her eyes.

Based in Chicago, Psychotherapist and the owner of Skylight Counseling Center David Klow, states, "women like direct men the same way a salsa dancer likes a good lead. When there is clarity and direction, she feels relaxed. If she can't trust his movements, they step on one another's toes. If he is direct and clear in his leadership, however, everyone wins."
Confidence is an asset that shines through in every facet of your life, and it is a very obvious asset (or an unfortunate lack thereof). Every woman respects a man with confidence because she is basically investing her heart and soul into a man who, himself, feels he is worthy.

Why Women Love Being With a Confident Man

1. **A confident, direct man will not waste her time.** A confident man will choose to be upfront and honest if he is not really feeling much of a connection after the first couple of dates, and he will have no problem being direct about how much he is into a woman when he does feel a real connection. The great thing about being direct is that a woman will feel assured that if something is bothering you, you'll be forthcoming and talk about it, which will put her mind at ease. If you are indirect and difficult to read, a woman will just surmise that you're not all that into her and that you're circumventing honesty most of the time. Even though a woman may be initially hurt by the truth, she would much prefer honesty over wasted time that she'll never get back.

2. **A man's confidence level shows her how he views himself**. If you don't have confidence in yourself, it may be difficult for her to have confidence in you

as well. Instead of nervously and self-consciously concerning yourself with the opinions of others, it's important to live your 5life the way you want to live it. Do things that interest you and make you happy. Seek out opportunities to explore. Don't hesitate or think, just dive right in. That is the only way you will be able to learn how to gain that powerful confidence that comes from living your life by your own standards.

3. **Confidence encourages positivity.** No one really enjoys being around someone who is constantly negative. Confident people usually think positively because they are secure in themselves and do not easily get thrown off track. Women love men who take life as it comes and react calmly and rationally in order to manage whatever the situation is and then are able to move on with fluidity. In other words, men who don't snivel or whine at whatever life hands them.

4. **The confident man does not cause her unnecessary stress.** Dating should not be stressful; it should be fun. It is difficult for anyone to trust someone who is indirect or ambiguous. When women

date these types of guys, it often results in the woman's confidence level sinking lower and lower the longer she has to guess how you feel or what you think. When you are really present with a woman, you are showing genuine interest in her, and that is what makes dating enjoyable. You should be able to make her feel secure. She won't want to risk getting hurt by playing mind games with unenthused guys.

Note: Direct dating coach Sasha Daygame, who authored "The Direct Daygame Bible" concludes that men being the 'mysterious type' only makes things more complicated and that playing at being mysterious only encourages awkward situations and complete inauthenticity. As an alternative approach to interacting with women, Sasha highly recommends his direct dating method. This method encourages authenticity, honesty, and expressing yourself assertively.

5. **The confident man is straightforward in his emotions.** A confident man has no interest in being ambiguous or unclear for fear of rejection. A confident man is emotionally clear and

opts to communicate openly about what he's thinking and feeling, rather than play at frustrating guessing games.

Chapter 5: The 10 Things Women Want Most in the Bedroom

Many men attempt to figure out what women are actually looking for and secretly desire in the bedroom, but unfortunately, many men don't ever really get it. Is she wanting candles lit for that ultra-romantic ambiance, or is she into having candle wax dripped on her nipples?

Would she rather be made love to very slowly, softly, and with feeling, or roughly from behind and with crazy mad passion? The answer is, yes. Yes to all of the above and more. What women want in bed isn't the same for every woman and what one particular woman may want in the bedroom can literally change from day to day or even hour to hour. Over 1,000 women were asked what they honestly and actually wanted from men in the bedroom.

Some of the results were things you may expect to hear but explained in more raw detail that makes the act make more sense. Other things that these polled women stated they'd like to have more of in the bedroom are quite frankly, shocking. These women got honest. They got real. And they got raw.

In no particular order, the ten most common things that women want most in the bedroom are:

1. **A woman wants you to undress her... slowly**. All too often, couples tend just to get down to business right away, and a whopping five minutes later, no one would never have guessed that couple was anywhere near being mid-coitus. Because of the (hopefully) raw passion of the 'wham-bam, thank you ma'am' method, it may serve its purpose for a quickie on many occasions. Seduction, however, is a dish best served slowly and methodically, and purposefully. Sex can be extra titillating – for both her *and* you – if you both just try to take your time unclothing each other. Reveal her body slowly as you let your eyes and lust wander, followed by your hands. Let them caress, brush, hover, and grip the places your lips and tongue will be sure to follow. **Men often complain that their significant other no longer wears the sexy undergarments she used to when they first started dating.** One of the biggest reasons for this is because men do

not take the time to appreciate the undergarments. The first time a woman goes out and gets sexy lingerie with her man in mind, and it goes completely unnoticed by him, it tells her that he doesn't really care about enjoying her in the way she has chosen to present herself to him. If you always strip your lady of her clothing in the complete dark, without regard to what she is wearing underneath, you really are selling your sex life short here gentlemen. Sex has many layers. While it's great when you get to the build-up of the climax, taking your time to enjoy yourself layer by layer can actually lead to a more exciting, fulfilling sex life.

"I want to be slowly unwrapped and revealed, like a present." —Debbie B.
"He needs to take his time with me until I can't handle it. And I want to   see him want me. It drives me crazy." —Michelle S.

The bottom line is that appreciation and anticipation go a really long way in making a woman absolutely worship you in the bedroom.

2. **Sex in public.** A woman may not want to go all the way and have sex in public (no

one wants to get arrested), but the draw here is the thrill of being observed in public. This is an enormous turn-on for many women. After all, as a teenager, we all were excited about the naughty things we did and never got caught, and that doesn't change completely in adulthood? Women love the thrill of you 'claiming' her in public in a sexual way, with anything from a kiss to...more.

Note: To the man who thinks his lady "isn't like that" - yes, yes she is.

3. **Role playing.** In a sexual nature, taking on different personas can be extremely liberating and may make room for thoughts and actions to be played out, which normally, you as a "real person" would not feel able to follow through with. By assuming a different role or putting on a costume, you can effectively kill off those inhibitions and insecurities that may otherwise prevent pleasure and sexual freedom.

"I love when he dresses up in his old Navy uniform. I didn't know him then, so it makes things different, and men-in-uniform really turn me on." —Jessie L.

4. **Let her take control.** When executed correctly, power has the ability to be a huge aphrodisiac for many people, men, and women alike. Just as with their male counterparts, at times a lot of women tend to like for their partner to be on the receiving end of the control. Even though most of the women polled were not looking for a BDSM lifestyle in particular, over half (53%) of those women were just as clear that they would like to have their partner to be involved in some type of submission, at least once or once in a great while. These women would like to tie a man up, spank him, and generally have access to every part of him. Another 9% of those women were interested in exhibiting the same power as a man. For these women, it wasn't enough for her to just be on top - they wanted the man on the bottom. Women have some of the same urges as men and would like the opportunity to express those urges, at least every once in a while.

"I really like being in control. Not every time, but sometimes. And I don't want to hurt him; I just want to do things to him. Things that please him, but also things that let him know he is not in control; I am." —Karen W.

5. **Make it all about her.** A woman wants to feel special, and a woman also wants to feel desired. When it comes to sex, men may think that some women are spoiled. There are many different ways and levels a woman can act spoiled, but keep in mind that she is also welcoming another human being to be inside her body. With that comes a combination of trust, submission, and comfort. As a man, it is imperative for you to invest the time it takes in order to make it about her by paying special attention to different areas of the body. Doing this will not only add to her pleasure, but she will also be more than willing reciprocate, so it largely benefits you as well. A little bit extra goes a really long way.

"I love when he will do anything to make me come. I'm not difficult, but that he wants it so bad is awesome!" —Fran U.

"I want him to look at me, directly into my eyes, especially as he puts it in. OMG." — Samantha D.

6. **A variety of motion and movement.** Over 80% of the women polled stated that more often than not they experienced men as having one speed: Way too fast. Woman after woman in this poll used these exact words to describe this quickness as "BAM-BAM-BAM-BAMBAMBAM!" That is actually exactly what these women said. Every single one of the women in this poll expressed that they enjoy sex more fully when there is a variety of types of touches and thrusts, and sex where the hands, mouth, and tongue continue to stay engaged. All of these women also expressed a desire for their partner to be more adventurous with his body position during sex. Women's bodies are really enjoyable and fun to explore. She wants you to experiment. Talk about what you are doing as or before you are going to do it and she will thank you in ways that will end up distracting you from work the next day, all day long.

"There are times I want him to go slowly, with love and affection. And other times I want it fast, hard, deep, and with aggression! I mean, just F*CK ME!" — Paula B.

7. **Take control**. Once the women who were polled finally let their guards down (yes, these women were protecting themselves or playing hard to get even in a room full of other women) almost all of them, 91% to be exact, agreed on one thing. As women, they wanted a man to take charge when it comes to sex and engaging in sexual behavior. This almost unanimous answer came from women from all walks of life, be it power attorneys, stay-at-home moms, women who are in their 50s, women who are in their 20s, corporate executives, emo girls, et cetera. Wealth, looks, upbringing, skin color, background, lifestyle, it didn't matter. The reason for this is excitingly simple - it's purely raw primal instincts. A heterosexual woman desires to be given pleasure from a man who is not only passionate and confident but also capable as well. Essentially, she wants to be able to finally just let go. She wants to be able

to trust a man enough in order to get a release, and just be a woman, unfortunately, many women seldom gets to be – sensual, sexual, and feminine. **A woman wants to be trusting enough to be able to hand the reigns over to a man who will not abuse her trust by using his "power" to degrade her.** Men who choose to do that tend to ruin the entire experience for the woman. Gentlemen, a woman who knowingly wants her man to take the lead during sex is seriously the ultimate gift. This tells a man that she trusts him with her body and the thoughts and emotions she may have during sex as well. **She is not only allowing him to take her; she deeply *desires* him to take her.** It is imperative to note here that a man by no means should allow that the control and submission in the bedroom should ever translate to a derogatory attitude of "she's my bitch" when out in public or around anyone else. Remember that being forceful and in control during sex does not mean being violent or angry. Before you try anything forceful or rough, especially if it is new, discuss limits and boundaries with your partner. This is where a safe word comes in really handy.

"I need him to manhandle me a little bit. I want to feel him want me. Put me against the wall and pull my clothes off." —Gina D.

8. **Foreplay. It starts *outside* the bedroom.** For many men, there are only really two types of foreplay – the anticipation of being touched and actually being touched. The thing that most of these men don't seem to grasp is that a man's version of foreplay doesn't usually include a woman's largest erogenous zone, which is her mind. There's absolutely no substitute for intelligent conversation and other mental stimulation as foreplay. For a woman, arousal often starts long before she may be consciously aware that it is happening. She may be turned on by a statement, by your wit, by a look, or even your willingness to hear her out without judgment. Seduction really is an art form, and it does require effort. Seduction demands that you focus on her. A woman wants to feel important, and she needs to matter, and she wants to feel desired. A

woman's biggest erogenous zone is her mind. Your words and actions as a man are the ultimate tools for her seduction and effective foreplay as a whole.

"He just starts. We walk in the bedroom, and he expects me just to flip on my back, automatically be wet, and ready for him to start thrusting." —Monica F.

9. **Go down on her - now and always**. About 75% of all women are never able to reach orgasm by penetration alone. That means if you're not going down, she may not be getting all she can be getting out of sex. If she wants him to engage his mouth in the Holiest of Holies, you need to value it and know what you're doing. You need to know how she likes it and when. Oral sex is a different level of intimacy. It creates trust when anyone allows another to experience their body so closely. That trust and allowance provides for an incredible physical and mental release, not to mention pleasure.

"I love when he goes down on me. Seriously. And if I get it first, it relaxes me SOOOO much, and I come SOOOO hard. Then he can pretty much have his way with me." —Joanne S.

10. **Kiss her - really kiss her.** Kissing is extremely intimate. From the first kiss on, kissing involves a closeness that is passionate, personal, and communicates a wide variety of things. Women often gauge the success of a relationship based on even the simpler first kiss. According to sociologists, there's a high amount of evolutionary biology, neurotransmitters, and instantaneous assessments of potential life-mates that all are products of the kiss. Generally, a woman wants a man to start kissing her softly and gently. Your mouth should wander as she gives you queues, so pay attention. Light strokes on the neck, face, and back will arouse more passion in a woman than kissing alone. When beginning to kiss, a light caress is strongly recommended, and should slowly give way to a firmer touch and grip as kissing continues and passion rises. **The timing here is everything. Kiss her cheeks, lips, neck, and**

eyelids. Take it slow. This will build her passion for you steadily and very strongly. She will get to the point where she feels like she simply cannot go on without *more* of you. Let it build naturally. Kiss her in the elevator, against the wall, in the shower, across the table, or in the car. Just kiss her. Be sure not to neglect areas of the body that often get overlooked, such as the inside of the wrist. This will slowly and sensually unlock her passion.

"Kiss my lips! Kiss the inside of my thighs! Kiss my neck! Kiss my hand! And please kiss me as you enter me when we are making love." —Michelle N.

"I like when he kisses me in public. I'm not one for Public Display of Affection, but to show everyone that he cares really special." —Betty C.

Chapter 6: The Campground Rule Revisited

In case you are unfamiliar with the campground or campsite rule, it is a rule that pertains to anyone engaging in a legal, consensual sexual relationship with someone significantly much younger and/or much more significantly inexperienced.

This could be an older man with a younger woman or man or an older woman with a younger man or woman. This rule gets its name from the idea that when you go camping, you leave the campground just like you found it or better. So in a relationship, this would mean that when the relationship ends, you would have inflicted any harm on the other person. You would leave them like you found them, or better.

We all have within us the ability to treat others well, to take the high road and respect the humanity of those around us. It is up to each and every one of us as individuals to make that choice for ourselves. Unfortunately, it probably would take you no time at all to think of an instance where you wish a partner would have and thought she should have, treated you much better than she did. At the risk of sounding overly idealistic, it is completely possible to adapt to the campground rule type of thinking in all of our relationships, men. Just imagine if every single person you've dated in your life lived by the campground rules. Would that affect you in a way that would change how you treat other people, namely women? Most likely.

Men naturally tend to take on more leadership roles than women. This being said while you're enjoying the benefits of masculinity, why not embrace a social structure that promotes the well-being of everyone, man, and woman alike. You're a man. Lead by example. Take the high road. Be a gentleman. Live by the campground rules. Show women that there are men out there who can be trusted. They, in turn, will reciprocate. So instead of a negativity begetting negativity kind of world, we could all choose to live in a world where we actively promote positivity begetting positivity.

We don't want any more soul crushing breakups after long, sweet partnerships. We do not need to be the guy that cheats on his partner; we can be the man whose partner trusts him because we do not give her a reason not to. Gentlemen, before we embark on our next relationship, let us make damn sure we know exactly what we are doing and already have a precisely clear path of where we intend on going.

Ways You Know You're Being Treated Well in a Relationship

- She inspires you to have a life outside of your relationship. This is a huge sign that things are going well and you are both on the right track.

- You have the desire to bring her home to meet your family. Introducing a woman to the family can be wrought with anxiety, but if you just can't wait for her to meet the folks because you want them to see what a lovely gal you've got, that meeting will be an adventure.

- When you experience moments of vulnerability, it makes you stronger. If you can confide in your partner about something that makes you feel a little jealous or embarrassed and they are there for you that only serves to strengthen your friendship and your love.

- She doesn't leave you hanging. Whether it's a date or your relationship in general, you know that she will come through for you. She is where she says she will be. She doesn't make you guess at what she's feeling.

- She makes you feel loved all the time. Every relationship has its ups and downs, but if she is dedicated to making you feel loved as a person and as a lover, you've got a winner.

Conclusion

Thank you again for downloading this book!

I hope this book was able to help you to gain a full understanding of what women want from men and what you want from a woman.

The next step is to take this new or renewed knowledge and put it into practice in your personal life. You will find that you are happier in relationships than you've been before, and the women in your life will respond to you with lasting honesty, passion, and loyalty.

Finally, if you enjoyed this book, please take the time to share your thoughts and post a review on Amazon. It'd be greatly appreciated!

Thank you and good luck!

www.ingramcontent.com/pod-product-compliance
Lightning Source LLC
Chambersburg PA
CBHW071326310526
45789CB00016B/1075